POETRY AND PREVENTION

POETRY AND PREVENTION

A LITTLE OUNCE IS WORTH

IRA E. HARRISON

To order additional copies of this book, contact:
Xlibris Corporation
1-888-795-4274
www.Xlibris.com
Orders@Xlibris.com
31367

CONTENTS

PREFACE

POETRY AND PREVENTION is the attempt of the author to become a more responsible husband, father and family member. It's the attempt of the author to become a responsible public health behavioral scientist. It is the author's attempt to not only practice what he preaches, but also to put it into print. It is written for children of all ages and stages. I often remind my children that their health is their wealth, and their wealth is their health!

Ira E. Harrison

ACKNOWLEDGEMENTS

I Thank my Wife, Claire Crooks-Harrison,

and my Daughter, Meri-Louise Harrison,

for reading and reacting to earlier

versions of this work.

ANGER (or It Felt Like What I Wanted)*

"It felt like what I wanted",
It was righteous indignation
When you dissed me—
Got me so blind—
Could not see or pee
So I tore into you . . .
Before I knew what I was doing
Stopped stupid like a punched out prune, \
It was not righteous indignation, but ANGER
And,
ANGER WILL EAT YOU UP!
ANGER IS AS REAL AS LIGHTING FLASHING AT MIDNIGHT!
IT CAN LIGHT YOU UP, LEACH YOU OUT,
ULCERATE YOUR INNARDS AND WIPE YOU AWAY!
YOU HAVE TO DEAL WITH ANGER: IT IS AS DANGEROUS AS DYNAMITE!
IGNORE IT AND IT WILL BURN YOU BADLY—SO GET IT OUT OF YOU: SCREAM, SHOWER, PRAY, DANCE, WORK, ROMANCE, WHATEVER, BUT LET
ANGER OUT FULLY,
GINGERLY BEFORE IT OOZES AND BRUISES YOU.
ANGER WILL EAT YOU UP,

IF YOU LET IT!

* ANGER eating *U* up is Unhealthy

1

AIDS*

AIDS,
Your deadly spell
Is everywhere—
WOE—
To he/she/it
Who does not care!

Sexually active people
Please,
Please remember these:
Abstinence, safer sex, and single partner true
Are the best live options open to you!

Sexually active people
Please,
Please remember these:
Abstinence, safer sex, and single partner true
Are,
The only live options open to you!

* Written in conjunction with PROJECT ALPHA: The Forgotten Partner, of the Education for Citizenship Committee of the Alpha Mu Lambda Chapter of The Alpha Phi Alpha Fraternity Inc., Mt. Olive Baptist Church, Knoxville, Tennessee, April 23, 1994; distributed in conjunction with PROJECT ALPHA: Teens Being Morally & Sexually Responsible, of the Education for Citizenship Committee of the Alpha Mu Lambda Chapter of the Alpha Phi Alpha Fraternity Inc., Community Evangelistic Church, Knoxville, Tennessee, April 29, 1995.

IF . . . (in the HIV/AIDS ERA)

IF,
You really have to do it?
STOP.

Think thru it . . .
Cover it—
Before;
YOU really, really SCREW it!

CPLOT IN SAN DIEGO

CPLOT* in San Diego
Was a journey strange
Geared to Community Planning
Leadership and change

Leadership in HIV/AIDS presentation
Problem solving, conflict resolution
And
Goals clarification.

Individual identification
Group process,
Cognitive stimulation
and eliminating stress.

Team building
And togetherness
Resources clarification
Reflection and rest.

Getting this together
For my CPG**
Will take a month
Or more for me.

However,
It is my endeavor,
And I shall remember
To share all this with the Tennessee CPG
In September.

* Community Planning Leadership Organization Planning
** Community Planning Group

ADDITION, SUBTRACTION, DIVISION*

You See

It always takes Two,

Unless there is One,

Who does not want to . . .

It always takes 2

Unless,

There is 1,

Who doesn't want 2

U C!

---

* *REAL* People Don't Rape*! Responsible Endearing Assiduous Loyal*
People Don't!

BRACES

BRACES OR SOMEBODY LOVES YOU*

Somebody loves you
I can tell
By the steel girders gripping your craggy teeth
As if to prevent a thief
Providing security against bleeding gray gums
Prophylaxis now
And for years to come
Against gingivitis . . .
Yeah,
You are loved very well
Awake or asleep
I can tell
Braces
Don't come cheap.

* Gladly having to purchase three sets for my children!

ADELE FAREWELL*

Adele Farewell

You know

I don't like goodbyes.

Deep beneath my eyes

Tears,

Carve Canyons of paralyzing pain

You'll never see—

Like the pain you mask from me.

Tears,

Flow silently out to sea

Buoyed up on some sunny shore

Where pain cannot endure

And rainbows swell

Adele, Adele, Adele

Adele, farewell, farewell.

* Written July 27, 1988 to my adorable stepdaughter, Adele Tyree, who died of cancer on November 12, 1988 at the age of 37, *CANCER & I met I 2 I and I have never been the same!*

CANCER+

WE CAN SIR
WE MUST SIR
FIND A WAY
TO CONTAIN AND CONQUEROR CANCER!

LADIES,
UNTIL WE DO
LIKE BIG ORANGE, MELLO YELLOW AND
MOUNTAIN DEW,
WE MUST SATURATE THIS REGION THIS
FALL
WITH PREVENTION AND TREATMENT
FACILITIES

FOR ALL,
Y'ALL
THAT'S ALL!

+ Poem written for the East Tennessee Coalition on Breast and Cervical Cancer's National Mammography Day Observance, Wednesday, October 19, 1994, Club Le Conte, Knoxville, Tennessee.

POETRY FOR NATIONAL BREAST & MAMMOGRAPHY DAY+

THE INVOCATION:
> Oh Great Spirit of Hygiene, Compassion and Human Understanding, Be with us as we meet, eat and consider the consequences of cancer for the families, friends and citizens of East Tennessee and all humankind.
> AMEN.

THE WELCOME:
> Today
> We are glad that you could come
> To be
> With us
> As we say
> "No Sir" to cancer
> "Yes Ma'am" We give a damn
> And shall continue to seek an answer
> To defeat breast and cervical cancer
> Until we do
> Preventative education will be our guru
> As we organize ourselves
> To see
> That East Tennessee
> Is aware of the latest
> In cancer
> Treatment, research and health care delivery.

+ Written for the East Tennessee Coalition on Breast and Cervical Cancer's Fall Luncheon, Calhoun's on the River, Knoxville, Tennessee October 25, 1995.

CATCHING A COLD*

Catching a cold
Can be the pits
The nose explodes
The head splits

The throat is cotton
The chest sweats
The body aches
The kidneys wet

Rolling in bed, from side to side
You're a rocking ship at ebb tide.

* Don't port yourself so fast that you comprise your immune system.

CRUD

This crud that has been going round
Thumps my throat
Syrups my sound
Reduces my range
Stenches me strange
Vetoes my voice
Gives me no choice
Such that I want
To pound the ground
And curse my fate
That I ought to be in this cruddy state.

DINING

Rather than
Eat to live,
We dine
To die . . .
Mushroom into
A Big Blue BALLOON
And,
    Wonder why???

DIET

ENOUGH

IS A FEAST.

TOO MUCH

MEANS OBESE.

TOO LITTLE

LEAVES A GREASE

IN THE BELLY!

DRINKERS*

Some drinkers are lovable, loud and lewd,
Like flypaper tied and tattooed;
But lawful, loyal and quite tame
Such that,
Even you
Treat them sane.

But others are loud, lewd, and crude
Like a spoiled, ugly, evil dude
Avoided, evaded, ignored as well,
With wild hair, wet body
Swaggering in foul smell.

Always *Be* *C*areful when *D*rinking.

DRUGS

Don't do drugs:
Drugs
Drag you

Down to

Death . . .

Don't do drugs.

DEATH*

Death
For the first time in history
YOU

Are no mystery

YOU

Enter and exit
Each night
Brilliantly
Like a comet's light
On TV screens, videos
                And

On many metropolitan streets, VIOLENTLY!

Always Be Careful, Death Can Wait—Make Death Wait!

DEATHSTYLE*

Walking death
Waiting to drop

Obese Beings

Unable to stop

EATING
DRINKING
CONSUMING

Unable to begin

Downsizing

Exorcism
                    Exercising.

* GET: Go Exercise Together!

EXERCISE: MUSCLE HUSTLE (1/19/04)*

Monday was Martin's Day,
Muscle Hustle got a bye,
Missing my workout partners
Made me almost want to cry.

Alberta, EP, and Lady Catherine,
Shirley, our leader, and Robert Chatman,
Nellie and Sara Lynn—
Even Mr. X, who 'as only just begun.

Well, Wednesday's coming,
And we'll see,
Who'll survive Martin's Day?
And Michael Jackson's calamity.

Working out, or in
With those you like or love,
Is a blessing from above;
Nothing to be taken lightly—
Thus I write,
This poem, politely.

* Working out regularly with proper mates is a worthwhile gait.

FLU*

TO THE ANGEL FLU (10/16/03)

> An angel shot me in my left arm,
> Saying this
> Will do more good than harm;
> Closing my eyes like I usually do,
> She said, "This shot prevents the flu."

* Fulton County came through for the seniors, me and you.

HANGNAIL (5/18/02)*

Here,
I hang at LAX, gate 52,
With a healthy hangnail
Not knowing what to do;
Can't borrow a nail clipper from an airline maiden
All because of Al Quaeda and Osama Bin Laden.

* A true occurrence in Los Angeles in 2002. Being healthy means that we must get a hold of ourselves, and leave not too much hanging whether hair, nail, or other parts.

LOVE . . . ANYTIME

LOVE ANYTIME
IS BETTER THAN RED WINE,
MORE FILLING
WHEN WILLING
MINDS, BODES RECLINE
WHATEVER THE TEXT:
TITILLATION OR SEX,
SHE'S REGINA, HE'S REX.

LOVE

LOVE! We all need love.
Like dry brown lawns need gentle rains.
Like the Earth needs the Springtime to give it zip and to
make it sing.
We all need love.
Love's touch,
Like the tender tapping of April showers sprinkles a balm
for our dreary hours,
Lifting our spirits, adding color, tone and buoyancy to
our being.
Love, like life dies without nourishment!
Love, unlike life requires both nourishment and
cherishment.
Yes! We all need love

MOLD (7/19/05)

Get a hold on mold . . .

Before mold gets a hold on you,
If you don't . . .
You'll end up black and blue.

Dampness and darkness
Stirs this slimy brew,
Get a hold on mold . . .
Before mold gets a hold on you.

Creeping down the shower door,
Creeping up the basement wall,
Reigning this dark sight to light
Before,
Your nose and lungs free fall.

IRA E. HARRISON

THE DRAGON*

> Addiction is affliction
>
> Watch what you eat or drink,
>
> The dragon,
>
> Once has hooked you
>
> (Has cooked you)
>
> Then,
>
> There's no time to think.

* THINK, about what you eat and drink!

DIET D&D

Dishonesty and Deception
Are some folk's diet,
It would make me sick . . .
I
Would never try it.

Decency and Dedication
Is more agreeable
To me,
Digestible and Delectable
Suiting me to a T.

NICOTINE, HARD LIQUOR, AND JOSEPHINE*

Nicotine
Is a fiend
It killed
My Josephine
Choke, choke
Don't smoke

II

Hard liquor
Chased her wine
They robed her down in pine
Think, think
Don't drink
Think, think
Don't drink!

* Before my former, became my ex, this was a timely and terrible text.

SMOKING*

Smoking was smart
When I was young,
But then
I was too dumb
To do it.

* Lettering in track and cross country in High School, I was not too dumb!

SSS*

Stop Smoking Son,
You're burning your innards:
Teeth, throat, and tongue . . .
Each puff
Is enough
To bring cancer—
A Disease—
To which,
Science has no answer!

* With my son in mind.

WOMEN AND WEED

I had the girls
The girls had me
Smoke was so thick
I could hardly see.

The girls are gone
And it hurts right here,
I can hardly swallow
A swig of beer.

SMOKE TRACK STAR

I dreamed of being a big track star
Slowed down,
Didn't get far,
Smoked a pack, or two
Coach said
I was through.

LOOKING GOOD

I looked good
With weed in hand
Cheeks puffed full
With weed from the can
And I could spit
A foot or more,
But my oh my
Did my throat
Get sore.

TOBACCO STAINS

Tobacco stains
On young bright teeth
May steal your breath
Like a deadly thief.

SMOKE

Smoke gets in your eyes
Goes up your nose
Fills the air
Presses your clothes.

Glides over the tongue
Like a deftly dancer
Into your throat throbbing . . .
May lead to deadly cancer.

STRESS

Stress kills
Don't mess with stress,
Exercise more
Eat less,
Enjoy life
Delay death,
Don't mess with stress;
Walk more
Talk less
Get rest
Pass the test
Live longer,
Without stress.

MESSING WITH STRESS

Don't mess with stress,

Walk a mile every day
Exercise stress away;
Prevent it from messing with
Work, religion and play
Rest stress at night
Dance refreshed by day.

TROUBLE

I have no trouble
Sleeping at night
Knowing
I've treated colleagues and students
Honorable and right.

Averted eyes
Evasive stances
Are absent
From my forward glances.

However,
There are those
Who,
Turn quick, look far awry—
Face frozen fast in Georgia clay-
With smiles on face
And hand extended,
Knowing full well
The relationship is ended.

- It's been said, Right don't wrong nobody!

WAITING ROOM* (12/27/04)

Emergencies,
Curled white, black, brown bodies
Bent towards the revolving door,
Patiently expecting to exit once more,
Less painful,
Upright,
All right,
And—
Out of sight,
But now,
Isolated,
Stabilized,
To be
Analyzed
Into medical care.

* Crawford Long Medical Hospital, Atlanta, GA.

SISTER, SISTER, SISTER LORETTA

It's never too early
Until it's too late,
Think wellness . . .
Drop the weight!

If you think . . .
Wellness is expensive—
Then . . .
Try sickness!

Keep the faith,
But loose the weight . . .
For your heart!

WITHOUT A HISTORY*

Without a history
You remain a mystery,
No one knows who you is,
Or were;
Whether you're
  Fruit,
    Fin,
      Feather,
         Flesh,
             Or fur.

Without a history
You remain a mystery,
No one knows who you is . . .
You fail the test
Miss the quiz,
Bubble
     Out into oblivion
       Without even
               A fizz.

* A holistic history helps maintain a healthy personality.

YOUR MEDICINE

Let me be your medicine

With dosage reticence,

Massaging mind and memory

From head to toe

With kind and careful chemistry,

Atomized love and energy

Lining lymph nodes with a learning and a burning

Blast and cast out

Sin, sickness and suffering,

No need for a prescription,

Aspirin, or bufferin,

No need at all

For Hadacol or Tylenol.

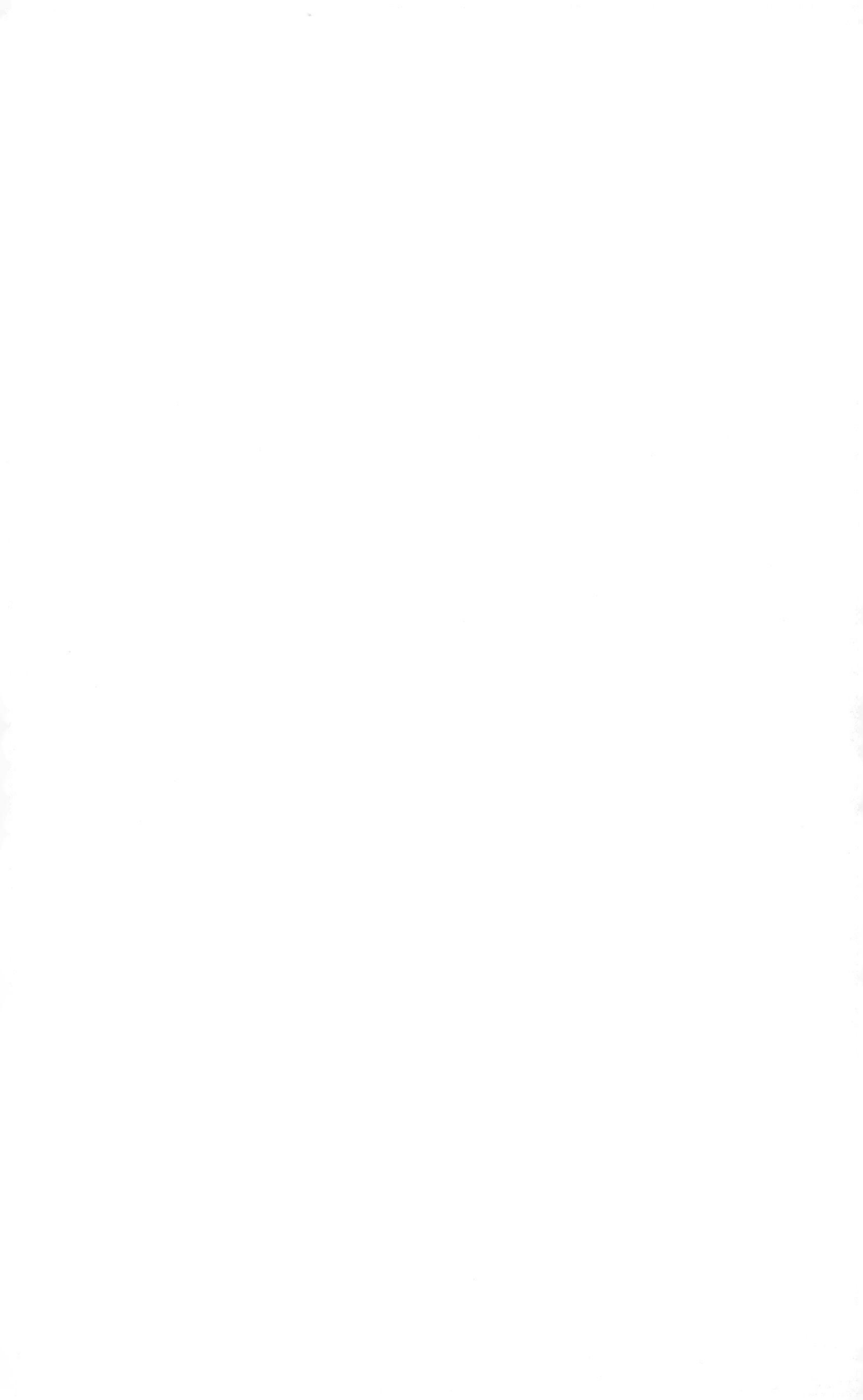